# CHAIR YOGA FOR SENIORS OVER 60:

## Instructions for Everyday Activities

JAMES BOWEN

# Contents

# DISCLAIMER

This book is as accurate and complete as possible. There may be typographical errors or mistakes in the content. This book also contains information that is only current as of the publication date. This Book is not the definitive source of information and should only be used as a guide. The book's sole purpose is to teach. The publisher or author does not guarantee the eBook's accuracy. They are not responsible for any error, omissions, or misinformation.

# HOW TO USE THIS BOOK

This book is meant to serve as a beginner's guide to chair yoga, complete with an introductory sequence. This order is based on my personal teaching experience and what I've found to be most effective. Class is structured as a whole and is meant to be done in its entirety. If you want to work on certain exercises on your own, you should warm up first.`

# WHAT IS CHAIR YOGA?

Chair yoga, also known as seated or supported standing yoga, is a gentler variant of traditional yoga. You don't need a lot of room or any specific equipment to practice chair yoga, so you can do it just about any place. Moderate stretching, self-massage, meditation, and breathing exercises are all viable options for chair yoga sessions and routines.

# SPECIFIC HEALTH ISSUES

## *Osteoporosis:*

To avoid causing damage to your joints, it's best to take it easy and be mindful when you move.

Gentle variations are best while twisting, and you should never use your arms to push or drag yourself into a twisted posture.

Forward bending should be done from the hips, not the spine. Imagine your chest is the leading edge of your forward motion rather than your forehead.

If at all possible, steer clear of bouncing or collision.

## *High blood pressure:*

Always have a level head and heart.

Take your time and pay attention as you go.

*Low blood pressure:*

Slowly regaining your feet after a forward bend (like in the Sun Salutation) might help you avoid feeling lightheaded.

# EQUIPMENT

## Clothing

Wearing clothes that are loose enough to allow you freedom of movement is ideal. Pants with an adjustable waist provide more freedom of movement, but a slack belt may achieve the same effect. Make sure that you are warm enough.

## Yoga mat

Putting a yoga mat beneath your chair prevents it from sliding around on the floor. When doing standing yoga poses, a yoga mat may also serve as a footrest.

**Block, bolster, and stool:**

Use props like foam blocks, a bolster, or even a tiny stool to elevate your feet and give them a rest. A steady object may be used to prop up your feet. A heavy book (such as a dictionary) may be used in a hurry, but a pile of volumes is not advisable since it might easily topple over.

**Chair:**

An armless, robust chair is ideal. Use a chair with arms if you have to, adjusting your postures as needed to accommodate them.

# SAFETY

**Using a wheelchair:**

You need to make sure the wheelchair is not tilting and that the brake is on before you start.

**Leaning against the chair**

If you're going to be leaning on the chair (for example, in a standing forward fold), you should either brace it against the wall or put the floor under all four feet (like a yoga mat).

# TIPS FOR YOGA TEACHERS

Students in a semicircle can all see what you're doing, and it fosters a sense of community and belonging among them.

Making direct, non-avoidable eye contact with kids has been shown to improve their ability to talk freely. Don't allow a lack of perfect chairs to prevent you from sharing chair yoga; make do with what you've got! There are a wide variety of suitable chairs (including dining chairs, couches, wheelchairs, and stools) that may be used for chair yoga. Use your imagination, but don't risk anyone's well-being. Watch out for seats that could be slipping. The chairs may be pushed up against a wall or placed on a nonslip surface such as a yoga mat if they are sliding on the floor.

# GETTING STARTED

**Grounding**

Sit in your chair with your hands resting on your lap or your knees. Feel the weight of your body on the seat and sense the chair, as if you have never sat in a chair before – how do your hips feel on the chair? Move your body gently from side to side and front to back. Feel how your feet touch the floor, bolster, stool, or blocks. Relax your shoulders and let your breath flow naturally.

**Basic sitting position.**

Blocks or a bolster may be used to elevate your feet so they can touch the floor while sitting.

**Using blocks to raise feet.**

**Using a bolster to raise feet.**

## MEDITATION

- Set a timer for one or two minutes.

- Relax your hands and shoulders.

- Relax and close your eyes.

- Become aware of your breath

Focus on the ins and outs of your breathing via the nose without altering it in any way.

- Notice if it is relaxed or strained

- Notice if the inhale and exhale are the same length

- Notice what temperature the air is as it comes into and leaves your body.

## BREATHING EXERCISE

This technique of breathing through each nostril in turn might help you relax and keep your left and right brain working in harmony.

This technique is called alternate nostril breathing because you will be using your right thumb and index finger to close off one nostril at a time while you breathe in and out (see pictures below). The right hand has often been utilized, although you may use whatever hand is most natural for you. The right hand is the one I'll be describing in this exercise.

When closing each nostril, do it lightly, using just enough pressure to prevent airflow. There shouldn't be any need to apply much force here.

- Sitting comfortably, exhale through both nostrils.
- Simply press your right thumb over your right nostril to close it, and then breathe in through your left nose.

- Drop your thumb and, while breathing through your right nostril, seal your left nostril with your forefinger.

- You should seal your left nostril and breathe in through your right one.

- Release the finger on your left nostril, seal your right nostril with your right \ thumb, and exhale via your left nostril.

Count this as one round. Begin with one or two cycles and work your way up to several minutes. When you're done, put your hands in your lap and take a few deep breaths in and out of each nostril.

**Hand position for alternate nostril breathing.**

# TRADITIONAL HAND POSITION FOR ALTERNATE NOSTRIL BREATHING.

The preferred finger position for alternating nostril breathing is seen in the first three images above. In the beginning, this posture may be more difficult for those who have discomfort or stiffness in their hands or fingers.

Explore both options and find which one works best for you. Regardless matter where you decide to practice this breathing method, you will get its benefits.

Make a right fist if you want to give it a go. Make sure your thumb, middle finger, and ring finger are all perfectly straight. Put little pressure on the fleshy region at the base of your thumb with your pointer and middle fingers.

Make the palm of your hand facing you. You may seal your right nostril with your thumb and your left nostril with the edge of your ring finger. Repeat the process of inhaling through each nostril in turn.

# WARM UP YOUR BODY

**Tapping and Self-Massage**

Method:

- Warm your hands by rubbing them together.

- Use a flat hand to tap, avoiding the joints, on the locations specified in the exercises.

- Apply light, even pressure while massaging the regions specified in the exercises that follow, avoiding the area around the joints and other sensitive areas like the belly and the face.

Precautions:

- Avoid tapping directly on joints.

- Massage with gentle pressure only.

Benefits:

- All over body warmth.

- Increases the circulation of blood to the skin.

- Relaxes the muscles and reduces tension.

- Heightens cognition of one's physical self.

- Boosts mental and physical performance.

**Foot massage.**

Raise your right foot and rest it on your left knee. Feel free to prop your foot up on a stool or bolster if you find yourself experiencing any discomfort.

Take a good look at your foot and see if you can see any changes in color or texture.

Beginning at the tips of your toes, massage your way down to your heel and then over the top of your foot.

Can you do the hand-and-foot clasp seen below, in which your fingers are interlaced between your toes?

Switch to the other foot and do it again.

**Foot massage on a stool.**

**Foot massage on a bolster.**

## CALVES

**Calf tapping.**

Use a flat palm to tap the whole calf gently.

Carry on for the length of around 5 deep breaths.

The process should be repeated on the other calf.

## KNEES

**Massaging the area around the knee.**

Feel your hands' warmth as you massage your knee gently.

Took around 5 deep breaths while saying this.

To do it again, switch knees.

## THIGHS

**Thigh Tapping.**

The whole thigh, including the rear, should be gently tapped and rubbed.

Carry on for the length of around 5 deep breaths.

Move on to the other thigh and repeat.

## BELLY

**Belly Rub.**

Gently rub your belly in a clockwise direction. Continue for the duration of approximately 5 relaxed breaths.

## ARMS

**Arm Tapping.**

Raise one hand and tap the raised arm. Keep your fingers away from the tops of your wrists, elbows, and shoulders.

Make careful to tap the inside and outside of your arm.

Rub your hand over your elbow, shoulder, and underarm.

Carry on for the length of around 5 deep breaths.

Switch arms and do it again.

## HEAD AND NECK

**Head, neck, and face massage.**

Do a slow, gentle massage of your neck, head, face, and ears.

10-20 easy breaths should be enough time to continue.

# CHEST TAPPING

**Collarbone and chest tapping**.

Just below your neck, on each side of your chest, you'll see two protruding bones called collarbones.

Tap your fingers softly on and around your collarbones, then down your sternum, the flat bone in the center of your chest.

Carry on for the length of around 5 deep breaths.

# HEART RUB

Rub the left side of your chest (over the heart) with a flat hand.

Carry on for the length of around 5 deep breaths.

# ACTIVE SEATED POSTURES

## 1. TOE RAISES

Method: You may rest your feet on the floor or prop them up on a bolster, block, or stool.

Raise your toes while maintaining your ball of the foot planted firmly on the floor.

Make a coiled motion with your toes.

Duration: Repeat 5 times.

Precautions: If you have a foot or toe injury, or if this motion hurts or strains your body, you should not do it.

Benefits: Improves blood flow to your toes.

Facilitates better foot motion and stability.

Boosts equilibrium.

## 2. ANKLE ROTATIONS

Method: Lift your foot off the floor and make circles with your ankle or for fun, try writing your name with your toes.

Duration: Carry on for the length of around 5 deep breaths.

Move on to the other ankle and do it again.

Precautions: Don't do this if you have an ankle injury or if this movement causes strain or pain.

Benefits: Increases circulation in feet and legs.

Improves mobility of the ankle joint.

Improves balance.

# 3. TOE POINT AND FLEX

Method: Raise your heel off the ground.

Your toes should be pointed.

Bring your toes up toward your shin as you flex your ankle.

Duration: Repeat 5 times with each foot.

Precautions: Avoid doing this if you've recently injured your ankle or if it hurts or strains your ankle.

Benefits: Enhances blood flow to the lower body.

Flexibility in the ankle joint is enhanced.

Boosts equilibrium.

## FINGER EXTENSIONS

Method: Raise your arms over your head.

Move your hands back and forth between open and closed fists.

Duration: Repeat 5 times.

Precautions: Don't do this if you have a finger injury or if this movement causes strain or pain.

Benefits: Increases circulation in the hands and arms.

Improves mobility of finger joints.

Improves strength in the muscles in the hands, arms, and shoulders.

## UPSIDE-DOWNSIDE FINGER EXTENSIONS

Method: Raise your arms over your head. Flick your palms up toward the ceiling and down toward the ground. Move your hands back and forth between open and closed fists. Invert your hands so that the palms are facing up and down.

Duration: Repeat 5 times in each direction.

Precautions: Don't do if you have a finger or shoulder injury or if this movement causes strain or pain.

Benefits: Increases circulation in the hands and arms.

Improves mobility of finger and shoulder joints.

Improves strength in the muscles in the hands, arms, and shoulders.

# WRIST EXTENSIONS

Method: Raise your arms over your head. Hold your wrists out so that your hands are fully extended and your palms are facing away from you. Bring your palms to your chest by bending your wrists.

Duration: Repeat 5 times.

Precautions: Don't do if you have a wrist injury or if this movement causes strain or pain. Benefits: Increases circulation in the hands and arms.

Improves mobility of wrist joints.

Improves strength in the muscles in the arms and shoulders.

## WRIST ROTATIONS

Method: Raise your arms over your head. Make a clockwise turn with your wrists. Counter-clockwise wrist rotation can help you.

Duration: Repeat 5 times in each direction.

Precautions: Don't do if you have a wrist injury or if this movement causes strain or pain. Benefits: Benefits the arms, hands, and shoulders by boosting circulation.

It helps the wrists move more freely.

Increases stamina in the upper body by toning up the arms and shoulders.

## ELBOW EXTENSIONS

Method: Put your hands at your sides, palms facing inward. Raise your thumbs to your shoulder blades.

Duration: Repeat 5 times.

Precautions: Don't do if you have an elbow injury or if this movement causes strain or pain. Benefits: Improves blood flow to the upper body.

The flexibility of the elbow joint is enhanced.

Adds muscular strength to the upper arm.

# SHOULDER ROTATIONS

Method: Place your fingertips on your shoulders. Make circles with your elbows.

Duration: Repeat 5 times in each direction.

Precautions: If you have a shoulder injury or if doing this motion hurts, you shouldn't perform it. Keep in mind that your shoulder should feel OK when you rotate your elbow. Determine whether there is a sweet spot for rotation when there are no clicks audible or felt in the shoulder.

Benefits: Improves shoulder blood flow.

As a result, shoulder mobility is enhanced.

Increases the stamina of the shoulder and upper arm muscles.

## SHOULDER RAISES

Method: Start with your shoulders relaxed and your hands on your thighs. Gently lift your shoulders up towards your ears. Relax your shoulders back down.

Duration: Repeat 5 times.

Precautions: Don't do this if you have a shoulder injury or if this movement causes strain or pain.

Benefits: Improves shoulder blood flow.

Boosts lymphatic drainage in the underarm lymph nodes.

As a result, shoulder mobility is enhanced.

Increases the durability of your shoulder muscles.

## HOLDING A TRAY

Method: Bring your hands in front of you with your palms facing up, as if you are holding a book or small tray. Gently move your hands out to either side.

 Duration: Repeat 5 times.

Precautions: Don't do if you have a shoulder injury or if this movement causes strain or pain. Benefits: Improves mobility of shoulder joints.

Improves strength in the muscles in the shoulders.

# SHOULDER SWINGS

Method: Position your hands low and in front of your hips, palms facing back. Put your arms overhead or higher.

Duration: Repeat 5 times.

Precautions: Don't do if you have a shoulder injury or if this movement causes strain or pain. Benefits: As a result, shoulder mobility is enhanced.

Increases the durability of your shoulder muscles.

# HEAD TILTS

Method: Start with your shoulders relaxed and your hands on your thighs. Gently tip your head to the right. Bring your head back to the center. Gently tip your head to the left.

Duration: Repeat 5 times on each side.

Precautions: If you have a neck injury or if doing this motion hurts, you shouldn't perform it. When moving, go only as far as you can without suffering any pain if you have osteoporosis.

Benefits: Helps loosen up the muscles in your neck.

Aids in greater neck flexibility.

# LOOKING LEFT AND RIGHT

Method: Begin by lowering your shoulders and resting your hands on your thighs. Slowly look to the right side. Keep your mind in the middle. Make a slow left turn with your head..

Duration: Repeat 5 times in each direction.

Precautions: When neck pain or strain occurs, you should cease doing this. Take extra precautions if you have osteoporosis. Don't forget that you shouldn't force yourself to do more than you're capable of.

Benefits: Stretches the muscles surrounding the neck.

Improves mobility of the neck.

## SKY AND SEA BREATHING

Method: Join your palms in front of your heart and let out a slow, calm breath. Raise your right hand and bring your left hand down as you inhale. Reunite your palms as you exhale and clasp them in front of your chest. Raise your left hand as you exhale and drop your right hand. As you let your breath out, clasp your hands again in front of your chest. Don't force your breathing; instead, breathe at a rate that is comfortable for you. Close your eyes and give it a go. How close can you feel your hands to your chest before they clasp?

Duration: Continue for 5 or 10 cycles. One cycle includes both sides.

Precautions: Do not attempt if you have a shoulder injury. Always go at your own pace and stop as soon as you feel any discomfort.

Benefits: Heightens cognition of one's physical self.

Has a sedative effect and helps calm the nerves.

Increases shoulder range of motion.

# HELD SEATED POSTURES

### *Gentle Twist*

Method: Have a seat. Begin by lowering your shoulders and resting your hands on your thighs. Put your left hand on top of your other. Turn your upper body to the left by gently twisting your waist to the left. Hold. Get returned to a neutral position. Hold onto your right thigh with both hands. Lift your right arm and gently rotate your upper body in that direction. Hold.

Duration: Hold for 5 relaxed breaths on each side. Repeat 5 times on each side.

Precautions: Do not do this if this movement causes strain or pain Remember to move slowly and mindfully. If you have osteoporosis, do the gentle variation with both hands on your thigh.

Benefits: Improves mobility of the spine.

Stretches the muscles in the back

## SIDE BEND

Method: Have a seat. Begin by lowering your shoulders and resting your hands on your thighs. Bring your right hand down to your side while raising your right arm over your head. Relax and lean leftward a little. Hold. It's important to have both hips firmly planted on the seat at all times. Get returned to a neutral position. In this gesture, the left arm is raised over the head while the right arm is lowered to the side. Hold. Alternatively, you might rest the palm of your raised hand on your head, shoulder, or even your lap if that seems too challenging.

Duration: Hold for 5 relaxed breaths on each side. Repeat 5 times on each side.

Precautions: Do not do if this movement causes strain or pain Remember to move slowly and mindfully. If you have osteoporosis, take a very gentle variation, bending only slightly to each side.

Benefits: Improves mobility of the spine.

Stretches the muscles in the side.

# SHOULDER STRETCH WITH STRAP

Method: Keep a belt or tie (a yoga strap works just as well) in your left hand. Hold the strap behind your head by extending your left hand straight over your head.

Put your left hand near your left shoulder and your left arm bent so the strap hangs behind your back.

With your right hand, attempt to reach behind your left shoulder and grab the strap, as indicated in the image.

Only move your hands in toward each other as far as you comfortably can without experiencing any discomfort.

Duration: Hold for 5 relaxed breaths on each side.

Precautions: Don't do this if you have a shoulder injury or if this movement causes strain or pain. Remember to move slowly and mindfully. If there is any pain in this posture, let go of the strap and return your hands to resting in your lap.

Benefits: Improves mobility of the shoulder joints.

Stretches the muscles in the arms and shoulders.


# STANDING POSTURES

## Forward Fold

Method: Remove yourself a foot or so from the chair and face the back of it. Suggested action: rest your arms on the seat's back.

Forward bending posture is achieved by maintaining the thighs parallel and the knees above the ankles.

Hold. Turn the chair around so that the seat is facing you if that's more convenient. Lean forward from the hips and rest your hands on the chair's seat.

Duration: Hold for 5 relaxed breaths.

Precautions: Do not do this if this movement causes strain or pain. Make sure your back and neck are straight. Always make sure you are moving slowly and mindfully, bending from your hips.

Benefits: Improves mobility of the hip joints.

Stretches the muscles in the back of the thighs.

## RAISED KNEE BALANCE

Method: You should face the chair when you stand.

Make sure your complete foot is resting on the seat of the chair as you bring the foot closest to the chair up to the seat.

Hold on to the chair's back for support while you strike a balance.

If you feel steady, try taking one hand off the back of the chair.

Duration: Hold for 5 relaxed breaths.

Precautions: If doing so causes you discomfort, you should refrain from doing so. Turn the chair around so you may balance on a stool or block if necessary. Remember to always walk gently and deliberately.

Benefits: Improves mobility of the hip and knee joints.

Improves the strength of the muscles in the standing leg. Improves balance.

## HIP HALF-CIRCLE

Method: Stand with your left hip beside the back of the chair and your left hand holding onto the chair.

With your right leg straight, move your right

foot: Forward and toward the chair.

Forward. Out to the side.

Back. Out to the side.

Forward. Forward and toward the chair.


Duration: Repeat this cycle 5 times.

Repeat the whole cycle with your opposite leg.


Precautions: Do not do if this movement causes strain or pain. Remember to always move slowly and mindfully.


Benefits: Improves mobility of the hip joints. Improves the strength of the muscles in the standing leg. Improves balance.


# TIPPY TOES

Method: Turn your back to the front of the chair.

Suggested action: rest your arms on the seat's back.

Boost yourself up onto the tips of your toes.

Test how silently and gently you can lift and put down your heels.

Duration: Repeat 5-10 times.

Precautions: If doing so causes you discomfort, you should refrain from doing so.

When you put your heels down, there should be no jolt.

Benefits: Improves mobility of the ankle joints.

Improves foot mobility. Improves the strength of the muscles in the calves. Improves balance.

## CALF STRETCH

Method: Arrange a small, folded towel on the floor behind the chair's back.

Stand behind the chair with your hands up and placed on the back of it.

Put one foot in front of the other with care, but do so.

The heel should stay on the ground while the toes are propped up on the towel.

Balance your body weight as you stretch.

Duration: Hold for 5 relaxed breaths. Repeat with your other foot.

Precautions: Do not do this if this movement causes strain or pain.

Keep the heel of the calf you're stretching on the floor.

Benefits: Stretches the calves. Improves mobility of the ankle joint.

Improves balance.

## SITTING TO STANDING

Method: When getting up from a sitting position, do so as slowly and steadily as you can. Get back into a sitting position. If you feel the need, you may use the seat for support or put out your arms in front of you.

Duration: Repeat at least 5 times.

Precautions: Do not do this if this movement causes strain or pain. If you feel very unbalanced, you can put a chair in front of you and use that to help you rise.

Benefits: The goal of this exercise is to be able to move from sitting to standing and vice-versa in a controlled way.

# FLOOR TO STANDING

Method: Stand beside the chair.

Use the chair to get down onto the floor, and into a sitting position.

Use the chair to return to a standing position.

The chair will be most stable if you keep the seat toward you.

Duration: Repeat at least 5 times.

Precautions: Do not do if this movement causes strain or pain. If you have tenderness in your knees, place a yoga mat on the floor where you will be sitting.

Benefits: This is a useful exercise for building the strength required to get up and down off the floor.

Working on this skill is critical since there are times when we may lose our balance and need to get ourselves back up off the floor.

# THE FINAL RELAXATION

Method: Relax your hands, resting them on your lap.

Let your whole body relax.

Close your eyes and pay attention to your relaxed breathing.

When you are finished; slowly open your eyes and wiggle your fingers and toes.

When getting up from your chair, do so slowly and in a controlled way to avoid dizziness. Enjoy the rest of your day.

Duration: Hold for up to 5 minutes.

Precautions: None, relaxation is suitable for everyone.

Benefits: Feels good. Calming.

Allows time for your body to start integrating the benefits of your yoga practice.

# CONCLUSION

I wish you well on your journey and am hopeful that this sequence serves as both a valuable exercise and a springboard for you to develop your own unique chair exercises. I'm thankful for the chance to spread the word about how wonderful it is to add exercise to one's life or to share it with others.